Nouha Farhat

Spinal cord ischemia

Nouha Farhat

Spinal cord ischemia

Imprint

Any brand names and product names mentioned in this book are subject to trademark, brand or patent protection and are trademarks or registered trademarks of their respective holders. The use of brand names, product names, common names, trade names, product descriptions etc. even without a particular marking in this work is in no way to be construed to mean that such names may be regarded as unrestricted in respect of trademark and brand protection legislation and could thus be used by anyone.

Cover image: www.ingimage.com

This book is a translation from the original published under ISBN 978-620-6-71721-8.

Publisher:
Sciencia Scripts
is a trademark of
Dodo Books Indian Ocean Ltd. and OmniScriptum S.R.L publishing group

120 High Road, East Finchley, London, N2 9ED, United Kingdom
Str. Armeneasca 28/1, office 1, Chisinau MD-2012, Republic of Moldova, Europe
Printed at: see last page
ISBN: 978-620-7-90434-1

Table of contents

INTRODUCTION

Spinal cord infarction (SCI) is both serious and rare. It accounts for 5 to 8% of acute myelopathies and around 1 to 2% of neurological pathologies of vascular origin [1]. Diagnosis is based on a suggestive clinical picture and magnetic resonance imaging (MRI).

Thanks to technological advances, MRI has become increasingly efficient, particularly in terms of diagnosis, thanks to the development of diffusion sequences.

However, the limited accessibility of medullary vessels for investigation remains a handicap in etiological diagnosis. This diagnostic difficulty is compounded by the scarcity and paucity of therapeutic guidelines, as well as a functional prognosis that remains poorly understood, with no consensus on prognostic factors, reflecting the unpredictability of evolution.

This pathology therefore remains a topical and controversial subject, hence the interest of our study to enrich the debate and better define this serious pathology.

The objectives of our study are to:

-Identify rare etiologies of MI.

-Updating the management of MI

-Determine the prognostic elements and complications of MI.

MATERIALS AND METHODS

1. Study description

This is a retrospective study including all patients followed at the Neurology Department of CHU Habib Bourguiba-Sfax over a period of 23 years and 14 years at the Neurology Department of CHU Sahloul-Sousse in whom the diagnosis of MI was retained.

We collected the clinical, para-clinical, therapeutic and evolutionary characteristics of all these patients.

2. Study materials :

2.1. Inclusion criteria

Patients hospitalized in the Neurology departments of CHU Habib Bourguiba-Sfax from 1992 to 2018 and CHU Sahloul-Sousse from 2004 to 2018 for MI.

- The diagnosis of MI was based on a compatible clinical picture in the absence of any other cause, whether or not associated with an MRI scan revealing signs of MI on sagittal T1 and T2 sequences, with axial T1 and T2 slices centred on the relevant floors. The MRI could also include FLAIR, diffusion and T1 sequences with gadolinium injection.

2.2. Non-inclusion criteria

Non-inclusion criteria included any anamnestic, clinical and/or radiological argument in favor of a differential diagnosis such as:

- Inflammatory or infectious myelitis.
- Medullary tumor pathology.
- Spinal cord vascular malformation (arteriovenous malformation, dural fistula, cavernoma, etc.).
- Hematomyelia

2.3. Data collection

Demographic and clinical data were collected from medical observations in each patient's hospital record.

Data collection included:

- Demographics :

* the patient's age at the time of the ischemic episode

* sex

- Clinical data:

*Personal history

* Clinical manifestations

* the semiological picture :

-Infarction of the anterior spinal artery territory

-Infarction of the posterior spinal arteries

-Brown Sequard syndrome

-Total transverse infarction,

-Centromedullary infarction

-Terminal cone infarction.

*level of injury: cervical, dorsal and lumbosacral

* selected etiology of MI

* the presence of vascular risk factors: hypertension, diabetes, hypercholesterolemia, smoking

* treatment

* evolution: data were collected from the follow-up medical records for each patient

Patient numbers are respected in the various tables and in the text.

Statistics

Results for descriptive data (demographic and clinical characteristics of each group) were expressed as mean with extremes for numerical values, and as percentages for frequencies.

RESULTS

We collated 19 patients who presented with MI between 1993 and 2018.

1. Patient demographics

The average age of patients was 53 (median 64), ranging from 13 to 81 years.

The population comprised 8 women (42.11%) and 11 men (57.89%).

Thirteen patients were hospitalized at CHU Habib Bourguiba in Sfax, and 6 at CHU Sahloul in Sousse.

2. Clinical data

The onset of neurological symptoms was described as abrupt and immediately maximal in 14 patients (73.68%). In one patient, the onset was a deficit noted on awakening. In 3 patients, the onset of symptoms was progressive, averaging 25.6 hours. The maximum duration of neurological symptoms was 72 hours in one patient.

The most common symptom was anterior spinal artery infarction in 16 cases (complete in 7 patients, or 37%). 3 patients presented a partial anterior spinal artery infarction (Brown sequard syndrome). Motor impairment was isolated in 4 cases. Sphincter disorders were of the retention type (7 cases). 9 of our patients (47.36%) took laxatives.

The onset was marked by acute spinal and/or radicular pain, which preceded the onset of neurological deficit in 7 cases. One patient continued to suffer from these severe pains on discharge from hospital. The deficit was total in 14 cases and partial in the remainder. 9 of our patients suffered from constipation, i.e. 47.36% were taking laxatives at the time of hospitalization.

Spinothalamic sensory disorders with a sensory level was revealed in (10 cases). Vibratory sensitivity disorders were found only in 3 cases.

Table I shows demographic and clinical data for all included patients (n=19).

Table I: Demographics and clinical signs of patients with spinal cord infarction

Patient	Age (years)	Gender	Clinical picture
1	50	H	Brown Sequard syndrome Sensory level D4
2	69	H	Interscapular pain Paraplegia Sensory level C5 Urinary retention
3	22	F	Interscapular pain Flaccid tetraplegia Sensory level C5 Urinary retention
4	64	H	Flaccid tetraplegia Spontaneous constrictive chest pain at rest radiating to the jaw
5	68	H	Flaccid paraplegia Brown Sequard syndrome Sensory level D 10

6	40	F	Flaccid paraplegia Sensory level D 6 Urinary retention
7	65	H	Flaccid paraplegia Sensory level D 6
8	13	H	Isolated flaccid paraplegia
9	81	H	Isolated flaccid paraplegia
10	63	F	Flaccid paraparesis Posterior cord syndrome Sensory level D 6
11	60	F	Retro-sternal burn Flaccid tetraplegia Sensory level D4 Urinary retention
12	71	H	Isolated paraparesis
13	20	F	Tetraparesis predominantly in the MS Cervical pain Cervical neuralgia C5-C6 Brown sequard syndrome

14	68	H	Isolated flaccid paraplegia
15	52	F	Isolated flaccid paraplegia
16	25	H	Tingling 2MI Flaccid tetraplegia Sensory level D3-D4 Urinary retention
17	78	F	Flaccid tetraplegia No sensory level
18	41	H	Lower limb pain Paraplegia Sensor level D10 Urinary retention

19	64	F	Upper limb pain
			Flaccid tetraplegia
			Urinary retention and cessation of matter and
			gas

3. Radiological data

Spinal cord MRI was performed in 16 cases. It was normal in 2 cases.

MRI was performed in the sub-acute phase in all patients, with a mean time to completion after clinical presentation of 48.35 hours.

A follow-up MRI was carried out in 2 cases in our series after 15 days and 3 months respectively from the onset of clinical signs (patient n'3 and n'6). In the first case, the initial MRI findings persisted, while in the second patient, spinal cord atrophy was observed.

The infarcts were located in the dorsal medulla in 12 patients (63%), the lumbosacral medulla in 2 and the cervical medulla in 5. Owl's eye sign was observed in 3 cases (Figure 6).

Involvement was centromedullary in 11 cases (Figure 2), lateralized in 3 and posterior in the remainder.

T1 sequences showed marrow swelling in 73% of cases, and a T2 hypersignal in all cases (Figure 1).

Diffusion sequences in 3 patients showed a hypersignal lesion with low ADC (Figure 3).

Lesion level correlation was found in 84% of cases.

Infarction of the vertebral body was observed in only 6 of 19 cases.

Figure 1,2,3 is the MRI of patient 3.

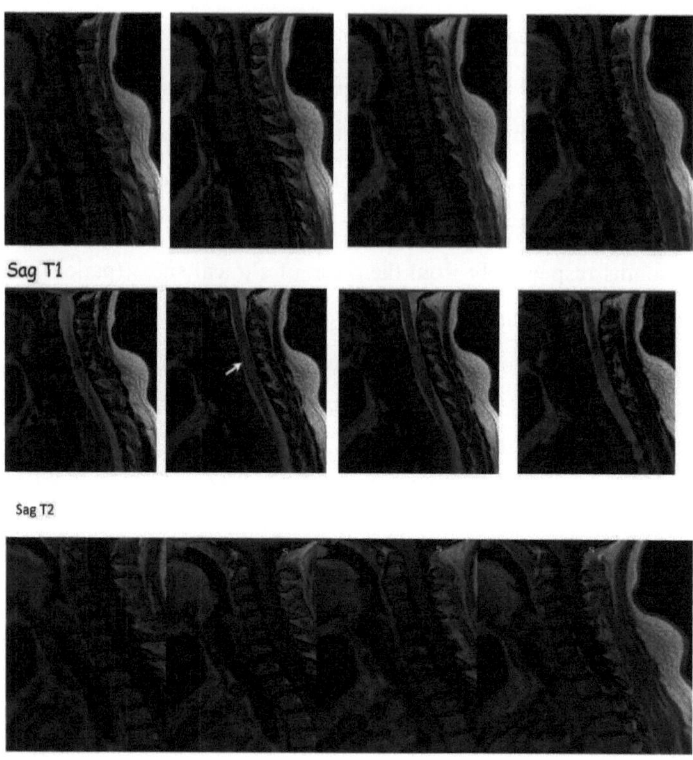

Figure 1: T1 i so s ignal lesion, T2 hypers ignal without extensive contrast pr i se from C4 to T1.

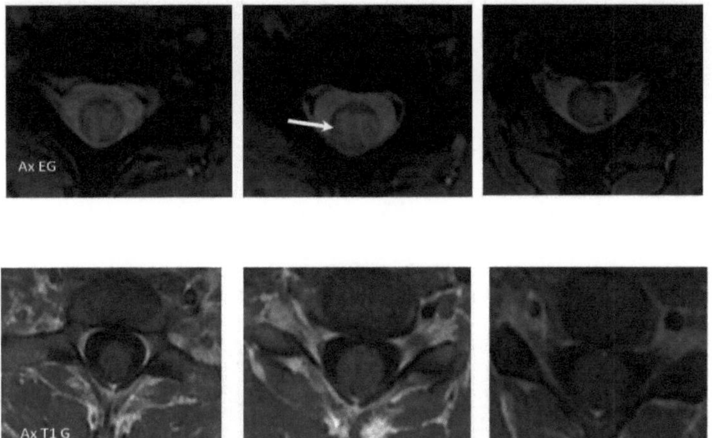

Figure 2: Spinal cord MRI axial sections Gradient echo and T1 with gadolinium injection showing a centromedullary lesion in T2 hypersignal without gadolinium uptake.

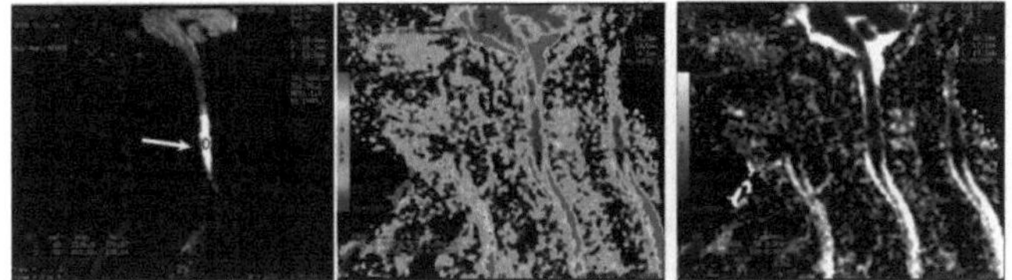

Figure 3: Spinal cord MRI sagittal section in diffusion sequence showing a hypersignal diffusion lesion with coefficient restriction of the ADC extended from C4 to T1.

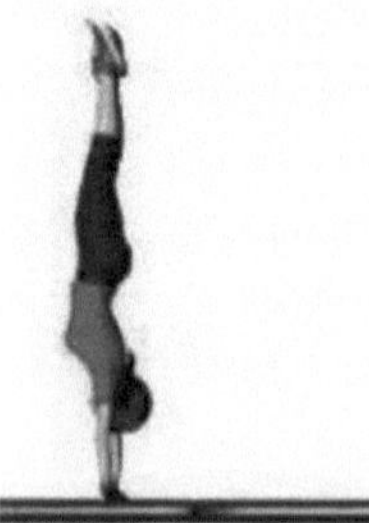

Figure 4: 4-hour training session for bac sport: reverse handstand

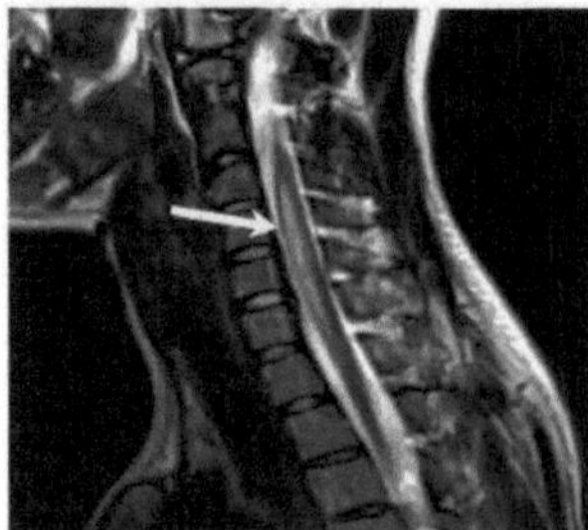

Figure 5: Sagittal section: T2 hypersignal lesion of C5 and C7.

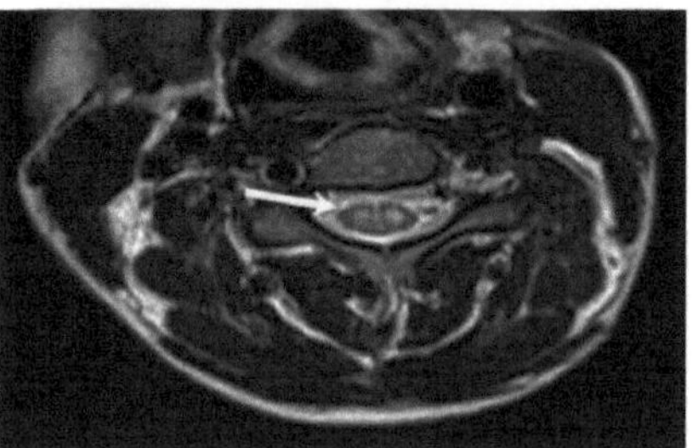

Figure 6: Axial section: T2 hypersignal with predominant anterior gray matter involvement, giving the appearance of an owl's-eye lesion (arrow).

Cervical IM on T2-weighted sequence of a 20-year-old woman who presented acutely, during a gynmastics session (training for bac sport which lasted 4H: upside-down handstand (Figure 4), flaccid tetraparesis predominantly in the upper limbs, intense and acute brutal cervical pain with C5-C6 cervical neuralgia. Neurological examination showed pyramidal syndrome of the lower limbs, sharp reflexes and Babinski sign, and right hemicorporeal spinothalamic sensory involvement. Deep sensory examination was normal. A workup including ESR value, C-reactive protein values and immune workup were normal. CSF analysis was normal. Spinal cord MRI showed a T2 hypersignal from C5 to C7 (Figure 5) with an owl's-eye appearance (Figure 6). Herpes 1, cytomegalovirus, toxoplasmosis, rubella, mycoplasma, chlamydia pneumoniae and Epstein-Barr serology studies in blood and cerebrospinal fluid (CSF) were negative. Visual evoked potentials were normal. TTE, TEE and thoracic angioscan were normal. The diagnosis of surfer's syndrome was accepted. The patient was treated with a 3-day bolus of solumedrol, followed by oral prednisone at a dose of 1 mg/kg/day. A partial response to the corticosteroid was noted (partial improvement of the motor deficit of the IM.

4. Etiologies

The etiological work-up was guided by the context and the presence of vascular risk factors. It was complete in 11 cases, including measurement of the SV, C-reactive protein values and immunological work-up, with CSF analysis and herpes 1, cytomegalovirus, toxoplasmosis, rubella, mycoplasma, chlamydia pneumoniae and Epstein-Barr serologies studied. ETSA, ETT, ETO and thoracic angioscanner were performed in the latter cases.

In the other cases, ETSA alone was performed on a patient with a history of cervical trauma showing vertebral dissection (Figure 5).

In the case of a patient with skin lesions suggesting herpes zoster, we performed ETSA, ETT, ETO and CSF analysis with the determination of anti-VZV antibodies in blood and CSF, without comparing the 2.

In patients 7 and 8 with hemodynamic failure, no etiological investigation was carried out, given the severity of the condition, and the diagnosis was made on the basis of the circumstances in which the motor deficit developed.

Table II shows the various etiologies selected for all patients. The most frequent aetiology of MI is atherosclerosis (n= 7, 36%), mainly of the aorta (Figure 10) or extending to all vascular axes (one of our patients presented on aortic and renal artery angioscanner with tight stenosis of the left renal artery, total occlusion of the right primitive iliac artery, pre-occlusive stenosis of the left primitive iliac artery >80% and occlusion of both popliteal arteries).80% and occlusion of both popliteal arteries.

In 2 cases, no etiology was found despite a complete workup. 7 patients had at least one vascular risk factor. The most frequent risk factor was hypertension (48% of cases). One patient presented with spinal cord ischemia caused by vertebral dissection (Figure 5). Other rare etiologies were found in our series, such as iatrogenic causes following interventional radiology procedures (treatment of abundant hemoptysis by embolization), vasculitis, whether infectious (viral) or inflammatory in the context of lupus disease. Spinal cord ischemia secondary to VZV infection was considered in an immunocompetent patient who presented with cutaneous lesions on the dorsal hemicepsis (Figure 10), IgM-type anti-VZV antibodies in CSF and dorsal spinal hypersignal on T2 sequences without gadolinium uptake (Figure 9).

The causes of medullary hypovolemia following acute hemodynamic failure due to MI with AVB or medullary hypoperfusion caused by compressive hemoperitoneum were noted in 2 patients. 2 patients, aged 64 and 81, presented with acute flaccid paraplegia following aortic dissection as assessed by aortic angioscan (Figure 6,7,8). Among the rare causes, we found surfer's syndrome in one patient following a gymnastics session.

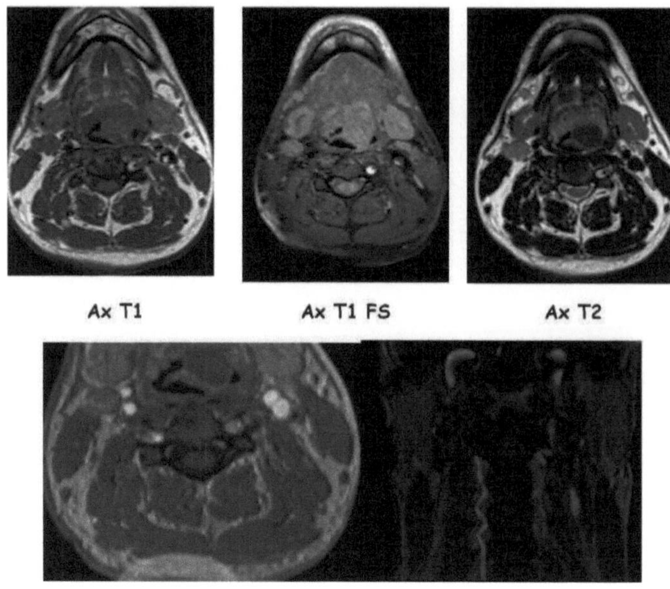

Figure 7: Parietal hematoma in the form of a crescent-shaped TI and T2 hyper-signal responsible for narrowing of the residual arterial lumen and string-like stenosis of the V2 portion of the left vertebral artery: dissection of the V2 portion of the vertebral artery

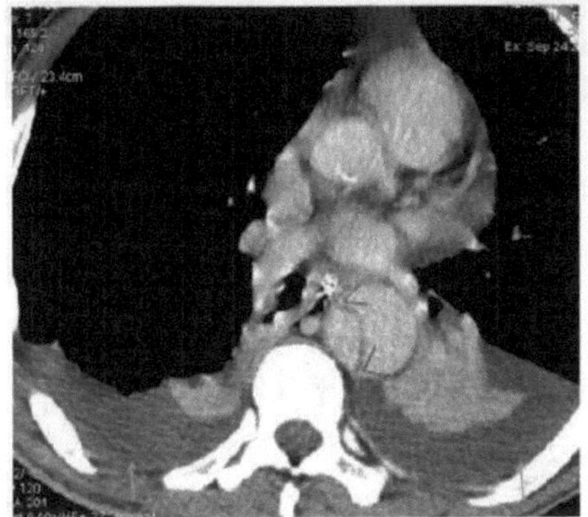

Figure 8: Axial section of aortic CT angio through the descending thoracic aorta in favor of aortic dissection

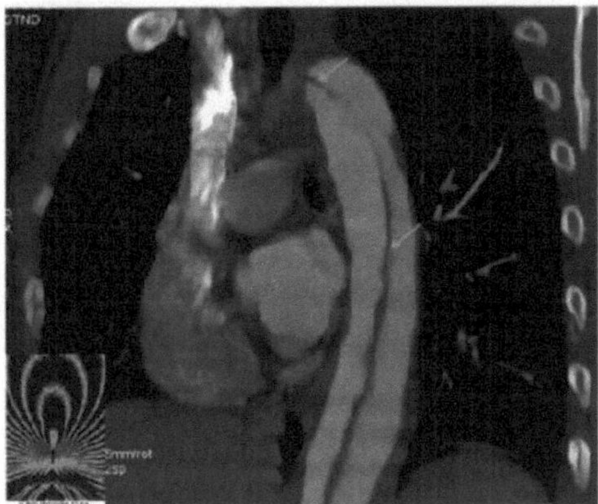

Figure 9: MIP sagittal oblique reconstruction of an aotic angio-CT showing an intimal flap

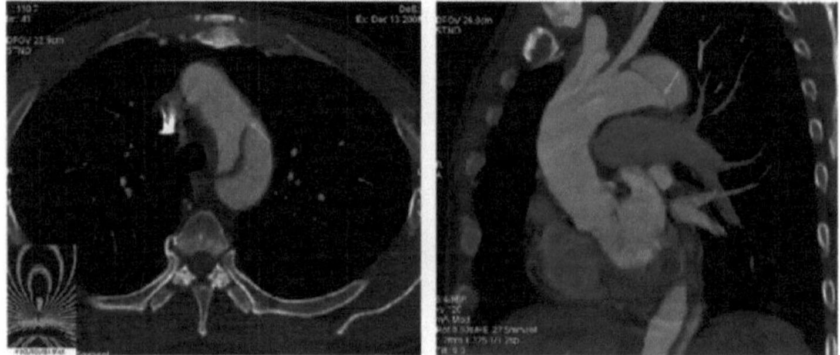

Figure 10:Axial section and oblique sagittal reconstruction of an aortic CT angiogram passing through the thoracic aorta: portal of entry of a dissection in a 64-year-old patient presenting with flaccid paraplegia and spontaneous constrictive chest pain at rest at 5 p.m. radiating to the jaws.

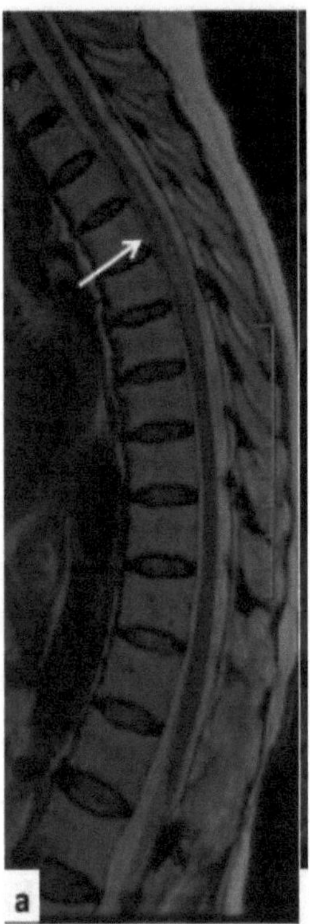

Figure 11: Sagittal section in T2 sequence showing a T2 hypersignal lesion in the spinal cord from D4 to D7.

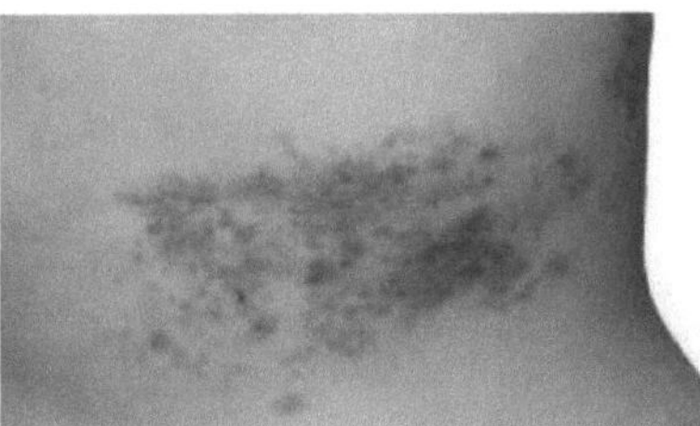

Figure 12: vesicular skin lesion of the thoracic hemi-girdle, consistent with a lesion caused by herpes zoster.

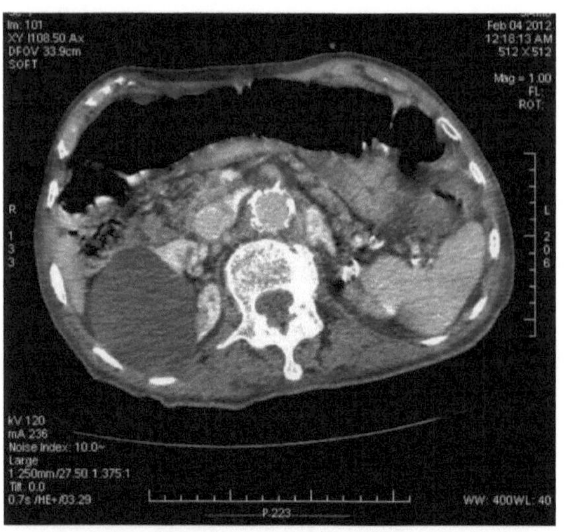

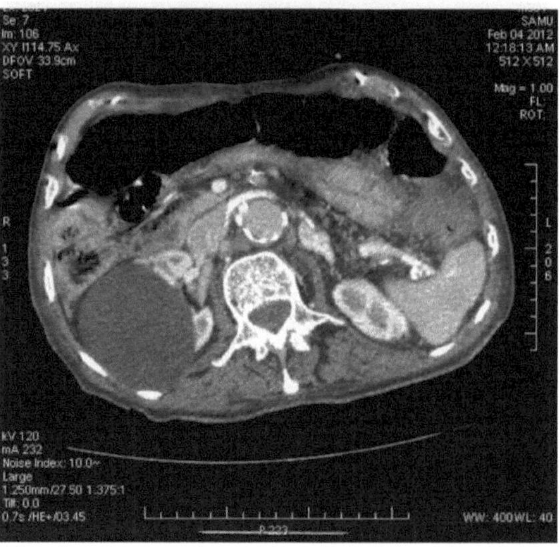

Figure 13: angioscan axial section showing atherosclerosis in the aorta

5. Treatment

Seven patients (43.75%) were treated with an antiplatelet aggregator in the acute phase of MI.

Curative anticoagulation was started in one patient following extracranial vertebral dissection, and one patient was being treated for pulmonary embolism. Six patients received intravenous corticosteroids in the acute phase at a dose of a one-gram bolus of methylprednisolone lasting between 3 and 5 days. The patient with hemoperitoneum received a blood transfusion to treat shock, and the 2 patients with aortic dissection were treated with antihypertensive drugs and analgesics. The patient with systemic lupus erythematosus was treated with corticosteroids, while Zovirax was prescribed for the patient with herpes zoster.

We noted a disparity in the therapeutic course of action depending on where patients were hospitalized. The team at CHU Sousse prescribed corticosteroid boluses in 5 of 6 cases, while patients at CHU Habib Bourguiba Sfax received antiaggregants in 7 of 13 cases. The use of antiaggregants was not correlated with the etiology of MI (**Table 2**).

Venous thromboembolism preventive anticoagulation was prescribed for all patients.

Treatment for neuropathic pain was initiated in a patient with persistent severe pain.

6. Clinical course and prognostic factors

Five patients (26%) died during the acute phase. The mean time from MI to death was 26 days (2-65 days). One patient presented with MI secondary to post-surgical aortic dissection. 2 patients died of hypovolemic shock with multivisceral failure. In one of the five patients, the cause of MI was undetermined, and autopsy was not performed.

Of the 14 survivors, 4 were transferred to a regional hospital. Finally, 10 patients returned home directly after hospitalization. The average acute hospital stay was 17 days. 31% were walking independently (**Figure 14**). 4 (21%) were continuing rehabilitation. Of these patients, 2 presented with 3rd degree pressure sores surgically treated by skin grafting, with good evolution. One patient continued to suffer from disabling neuropathic pain, requiring treatment with carbamazepine, pregabalin and a tricyclic antidepressant without improvement. Vesico-sphincter disorders required intermittent urinary catheterization in 2 patients. Gender did not influence the course of MI. Early age was a good prognostic factor. We found a correlation between the size of the initial motor deficit and the degree of recovery of the motor deficit, as well as the cause of the MI. Among the 7 patients with vesico- sphincter disorders, 2 remained bedridden. We found no correlation between initial clinical symptoms (pain) and neurological examination findings (presence or absence of deep sensory involvement or sensory level), the territory of involvement and the prognosis of the pathology. We also found no correlation between MRI appearance (sagittal or axial location of lesion, extent of lesion) and disease prognosis. Etiology was the only prognostic factor. Patients with either infectious or immune vasculitis responded well to treatment, as did the 2 cases of vertebral dissection and surfer's syndrome.

The evolution of MI caused by atherosclerosis was unpredictable.

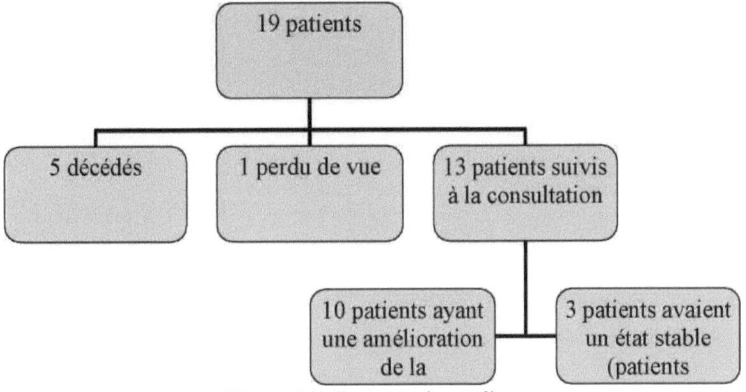

Figure 14: Patient chart flow

P	Etiology	Treatment	Evolution
1	Interventional radiology procedures (treatment of profuse hemoptysis by embolization)	Carbamazepine, Rivotril, Anafranil, Pregabalin	Persistence of disabling neuropathic pain Autonomous walking
2	Vasculopathy secondary to VZV infection	Zovirax (10mg/kg/8H) X 21 days Methylprednisolone (1 g/d X 3 days	Partial improvement of motor deficit Independent walking
3	Spinal dissection	Anticoagulant	Partial improvement in deficit 2 MS engines Stable
4	Aortic dissection (Figure 10)	Analgesic Antihypertensive	
5	Atherosclerosis	Anti-aggregants (Aspirin)	
6	Systemic lupus erythematosus	Anti-aggregants (Aspirin) Corticosteroid therapy	Improvement Independent walking
7	Acute hemodynamic failure due to a IDM with BAV	Antiaggregants (Aspirin, Plavix)	Deaths
8	Medullary hypoperfusion following hemo compressive peritoneum	Blood transfusion Treatment of hemorrhagic shock and hemoperitoneum	Deaths
9	Dissection of the aorta	Antihypertensive treatment	Deaths
10	Atherosclerosis	Antiaggregant	Improvement
11	Atherosclerosis	Antiaggregant	Independent walking Stable
12	Atherosclerosis	Antiaggregant	Improvement

13	Surfer's syndrome	Methylprednisolone (1g/d X 5d)	Independent walking Improvement
14	(gymnastics session)		Independent walking
15	Undetermined Atherosclerosis	- Antiaggregant	Deaths Improvement of motor deficit in
16	Undetermined		10 days
17	Atherosclerosis	- Methylprednisolone (1g/d X 5d)	Recovery of motor deficit in the 2 MS Moderate MI deficit persists in 1 month Deaths
18	Atherosclerosis	Methylprednisolone (1g/d X 5d)	Improving the motor skills of a
19	Undetermined	Methylprednisolone (1g/d X 5d)	side. Unable to walk at 1 month Partial improvement in deficit engine in 25J

DISCUSSION

1. Demographics

The mean age of our population is comparable to that of populations in the literature, ranging from 54 years in the de Sèze et al. team to 73 years in the Kumral et al. study ([1], [2]).

The sex ratio differs from one study to another, but 7 studies find, as we do, a male predominance of MI [3].

No explanation has been put forward to explain this male predominance. The importance of atheromatous origin of MI in our study could be a hypothesis explaining this male overrepresentation, male sex being a vascular risk factor. However, this predominantly atheromatous origin is not found in other studies identifying a male predominance [3].

2. Clinical symptoms

The most common symptom in all studies, including our own, is involvement of the anterior spinal artery territory ([4], [5]). The fragility of the anterior spinal artery territory is explained by the uniqueness of this artery, and by the smaller number of radiculo-medullary arteries irrigating its thoracic portion, compared with the posterior spinal arteries. Indeed, as in our study, these MI tend to be located most often in the lower thoracic segment of the medullary cord [6]. These infarcts generally present with severe pain at the same level as the infarct, and with superficial sensory impairment below the site of the MI [7].

Functional impairment in our patients appears to be similar in intensity to that reported in the literature. Indeed, 14 patients, or 73% of our population, present a total deficit in the acute phase, whereas in the literature this intensity is found between 42% and 75% of the populations described

([1], [4]). This may be linked to a similar proportion of patients with anterior spinal artery involvement in our population (84% in our series, compared with 72.7% for Cheng et al. [8]).

Nearly half of our patients (7 patients or 37%) had a urinary catheter in the acute phase of MI. Compared with the 90 literature, our population had a lower frequency of sphincter disorders. Indeed, the need for a urinary catheter was present in 79.8% of patients in Robertson et al. and 54% of patients in New et al ([3], [9]).

The symptomology of vesico-sphincter disorders depends on the level of spinal cord injury and whether or not the sympathetic and para-sympathetic vegetative systems are affected. Concerning the use of laxatives, 9 of our patients (47.36%) consumed them. In the study by New et al. 33 patients (77%) were taking laxatives at discharge, and 2 patients (5%) were anal incontinent [9]. Constipation in spinal cord injury is linked to damage to extrinsic innervation, resulting in loss of colonic control, with anal incontinence or constipation often associated in these patients [10]. Our patients therefore suffer less damage to the urinary and digestive systems during hospitalization than those reported in the literature.

In our study, 7 out of 19 patients (36.84%) experienced pain during acute hospitalization. Acute-phase pain with a frequency ranging from 32 to 72% of patients ([2], [3], [8]). Our results were similar to those of the Kumral et al., Cheng et al. and Novy et al. series, with only one patient not experiencing spontaneous pain relief during hospitalization ([2], [7], [8]). Indeed, in the acute phase of our study, only one of the 7 patients had severe pain at discharge.

3. Radiological signs

Investigations of MI must include spinal cord MRI. However, in the presence of a typical clinical picture, radiological confirmation is not necessary to establish the diagnosis. The contribution of imaging is essential to exclude other differential diagnoses, particularly compression of the ME. MRI can also be useful in differentiating MI from other vascular disorders (dural arteriovenous fistula) or inflammatory myelitis. In the latter case, lumbar puncture is recommended to exclude an inflammatory cause when the clinical picture is suggestive. In MI, authors have reported the presence of a T2 and FLAIR hypersignal lesion, generally in the central part of the medulla. Vargas et al illustrated the advances made in imaging for the exploration of ME. They emphasized that diffusion sequences are the key sequences in MI, showing a diffusion hypersignal with decreased ADC coefficient without gadolinium uptake [11]. This anomaly appears in the sub-acute phase, as in our study. Its sensitivity is much lower in the spinal cord than in the brain, due to the risk of image artifacts caused by narrow channels [12]. Occasionally, there may be vertebral body infarcts associated with ME infarcts, as in 6 cases in our study, since these 2 anatomical structures are vascularized by intercostal arteries [12]. These features are seen in the subacute phase. As the infarction becomes more chronic, the ME atrophies and myelomalacia appears, which was observed on a control MRI performed on one of our patients at 3 months. Infarcts of the anterior spinal artery can take on the appearance described in 3 cases in our study as "owl's eyes" or "snake eyes" on axial sections of T2-weighted images, due to the presence of bilateral hypersignal of the anterior horn of the gray matter [4]. T1 sequences may be normal or show swelling of the ME and moderate hypersignal of the medullary cord. All these aspects were revealed in 73% of cases in our study.

4. Etiologies

As part of the etiological assessment, bone imaging plays a vital role in the absence of an obvious iatrogenic cause. Angioscan of ASD can be performed to look for vertebral artery dissection. In dorsal or conus medullaris MI, thoracoabdominal angioscanning has been shown to be useful in the search for an aneurysm or aortic dissection. Echocardiography is mandatory as part of the etiological investigation in search of endocarditis or intracavitary thrombus, and TEE enables visualization of the proximal aorta, revealing upper aortic dissection, aneurysm or atherosclerosis. A thrombophilia work-up should be considered in young patients in the absence of vascular risk factors. An immunoassay and lumbar puncture are indicated if vasculitis is suspected. Marrow angiography is recommended if the etiological work-up remains negative. It can show vascular malformation (arteriovenous malformation or dural arteriovenous fistula), as this could explain ME ischemia due to venous congestion or occlusion of the anterior spinal artery [15]. However, in the case of MI with a clear arterial distribution, the yield of spinal angiography remains low.

The etiologies of MI are multiple and variable in the literature. This variability is probably a function of the mode of recruitment (rehabilitation department, post-aortic surgery patients, neurology department, etc.). Only the proportion of patients with an undetermined cause remains stable at around 20% in these studies, and 10% in our study [4].

The most common risk factor in our population (48%) was hypertension, in line with the majority of MI studies ([7], [16]). Only the study by Kumral et al. found smoking to be the most frequent risk factor, immediately followed by hypertension [2]. The most frequently identified etiology is damage to the aorta [20]. The causes of this damage in adults are atherosclerosis [20], cardiac surgery [17], aortic rupture following trauma, spontaneous rupture of aneurysms and thrombosis. MI following surgery on a thoracoabdominal aortic aneurysm is by far the most frequent cause [21]. Degenerative complications of the cervical spine with compression of the radicular artery can cause MI. Other etiologies include traction for scoliosis after orthopaedic surgery [18], complications of cardiac surgery and sickle cell disease [19].

Vertebral artery dissection has also been identified as a cause of MI, the most common location being C2-C5 [22]. In a meta-analysis, 1.8% of patients with vertebral artery dissection had associated cervical myelopathy [23]. These patients most often presented with posterior cord syndrome or Brown sequard syndrome [22].

Surfer's myelopathy was among the rare causes identified in our series. 64 cases suffering from this pathology have been described in the literature [24]. The diagnosis of non-traumatic MI, termed surfer's myelopathy in a gymnast was retained among these cases. The clinical manifestations and MRI appearance in our patient were similar to those reported in the literature of Surfer's myelopathy [25, 26]. This underlines the importance of physician and patient awareness of this rare disease. There are many pathophysiological hypotheses for these pathologies, the most widely adopted being that of vasospasm caused by perforation of the radicular vessels following prolonged hyperextension of the head, or by the presence of fibrocartilaginous emboli [27].

The diagnosis of MI secondary to VZV vasculitis was made on the basis of an acute onset of medullary syndrome associated with vesicular lesions of herpes zoster skin, or on the basis of viral serology even in the absence of such lesions. Diagnostic confirmation, prior to the development of diffusion sequence MRI, was based on post-mortem anatomopathological studies of ME necrosis secondary to VZV vasculitis. Today, diffusion MRI is used in conjunction with the search for intrathecal anti-VZV IgG synthesis to support the diagnosis of post-VZV MI (the ratio of anti-VZV IgG antibody level in serum/low anti-VZV IgG antibody level in CSF) [28].

5. Treatment

Given the rarity of this condition and the multitude of etiologies involved, guidelines are few and far between, and therapeutic research remains limited. There have been no major clinical trials examining the efficacy of these treatments. In a recent study, the authors stressed the importance of increasing spinal cord blood flow. Otherwise, treatment is generally guided by the etiology of the MI [28]. Vertebral artery dissection, as in our case, should be treated with anticoagulants. In the absence of etiology in a patient with atherosclerosis in other vascular territories, treatment is based on control of vascular risk factors, as in our study (hypertension, diabetes, statins and antiplatelet agents).

In the acute phase, there are a few case reports showing the benefit of IV thrombolysis for this condition [29-32]. There are no published studies to date on the use of IV thrombolytic therapy in patients with MI. However, there is an ongoing clinical trial examining the safety and efficacy of IV thrombolytics in patients with anterior spinal artery infarcts hospitalized within 6 h of symptom onset (NCT02242084). Certain contraindications are specific to MI, such as aortic dissection, bleeding in the ME, arteriovenous malformations or spinal cord compression by a tumor.

According to the latest recommendations, new therapeutic options are being implemented, such as the use of vasopressors and CSF drainage to increase ME perfusion. These are not part of the therapeutic arsenal used in our study.

These external CSF drains would be placed peri-operatively and immediately after ME surgery or endovascular treatment of a thoracic aortic aneurysm, and removed after 72 h [33, 34]. They reduce CSF pressure and resistance to blood flow in the spinal arteries, thereby increasing ME perfusion [35]. A randomized clinical trial is currently underway to study the benefit of using CSF drainage in patients with MI following aortic aneurysm surgery. Drainage complications would be multiple but controllable: direct nerve damage or hematomas following drain placement, infections, and intracranial hypotension leading to headache and subdural hematoma [36]. There are no published studies on the use of CSF drainage for other etiologies of MI.

Vasopressors may increase ME perfusion pressure through collaterals [37].

In the absence of these therapeutic options, treatment generally involves controlling risk factors whenever possible with antithrombotic therapies (antiplatelet or anticoagulant) and controlling vascular risk factors (hypertension, diabetes).

There are few treatments that could be adapted to the etiology. For example, vertebral artery dissection should be treated with an antiplatelet agent or anticoagulation. In the case of vasculitis, corticosteroids and immunomodulators are generally indicated [33, 34]. This was our therapeutic approach in cases of vasculitis and dissection. The use of corticosteroids is not recommended in patients with MI unrelated to vasculitis. In fact, it makes sense to limit our prescription of corticosteroids in other etiologies.

Prescription of statins or antihypertensives is more frequent in our group of patients. These two treatments reflect an atheromatous background and may act on the aortic atherosclerosis in question. In our study, the most frequently used analgesics were antiepileptics, probably by analogy with the management of post-traumatic spinal cord pain [3].

6. Prognosis

Several studies have reported reduced life expectancy in patients with MI [3,38, 39].

In our study, 5 patients died (26%). In the literature, mortality ranges from 4.5% to 30% [3, 38, 39]. Our figures are therefore comparable to those found in other studies of MI.

MI secondary to aortic dissection is associated with a high mortality rate compared with those without MI [40]. One patient in our study with aortic dissection died and the other remained bedridden. In a study of 25 cases, iatrogenic MI showed slight improvement at follow-up in 50% of cases. In 25% of cases, no improvement was observed and 25% had almost complete recovery of the motor deficit [40]. Our patient who presented with MI following an interventional radiology procedure (treatment of profuse hemoptysis by embolization) recovered well, retaining only intense neuropathic pain. Poor prognostic factors included severe impairment in the acute phase (total deficit, vesico-sphincter disorders, or proprioceptive impairment), female gender, elderly subject and lack of improvement within the first hour 24 [16,42]. In our study, the extent of motor deficit, advanced age, etiology and lack of recovery in the acute phase were correlated with a poor prognosis. We found no association between gender, presence of vesico-sphincter disorders and posterior cord involvement with prognosis.

However, it should be stressed that improvement can be observed even years after the incident with regular rehabilitation. One study showed that, following long-term follow-up, 41% of wheelchair-bound patients in hospital had regained their ability to walk, and 33% of patients requiring bladder catheterization in hospital improved [43,44]. These same findings were revealed in our study. Long-term follow-up studies report pain in 31% to 70% of patients [3]. In our study, only one patient retained disabling pain.

The good recovery after MI could be explained by a certain neuronal plasticity observed by studies [45, 46].

Studies of long-term follow-up in MI focus on clinical and functional recovery. In our study, the functional evolution of our patients was favorable, since at the 6-month follow-up visit, 6 patients (31%) were walking independently and 89% had normal vesico-sphincter function. In the literature, patients had autonomous walking in 8 to 41% of cases remote from the infarction [47], [48]. Thirty-one to 55% of patients used an indwelling or intermittent urinary catheter [48]. Vesico- sphincter disorders required intermittent urinary catheterization in 2 of our patients. Our study did not include data on erectile dysfunction. In the literature, we found only one study dealing with erectile dysfunction after MI, which reported 3 cases of erectile dysfunction, including two cases of impotence, out of 44 MI cases [49].

Unfortunately, there are few studies comparing the prognosis of MI with that of other spinal cord injuries. In these studies, a comparison of populations with ischemic or traumatic spinal cord injury shows that patients with MI are older and more often female. However, there was no difference in functional prognosis **[50-53].**

7. Study limits

As with any study, our investigation had a number of methodological limitations. The number of patients was small, despite the fact that we recruited from 2 university hospitals over a long period. This may be explained by the rarity of this pathology.

To complete the analysis, we need to call on other Tunisian and even North African neurology centers.

CONCLUSION

MI frequently affects the lower part of the dorsal ME. Diffusion MRI was the most effective means of retaining the diagnosis of MI.

Our study highlighted rare etiologies of MI such as surfer's myelopathy, systemic lupus erythematosus, post VZV vasculitis.

Other exceptional causes have been reported in the literature, such as Scheuermann's disease, a skeletal growth disorder of the vertebrae causing spinal deformity in the form of kyphosis and consequent compression of the circumferential arteries and MI [54], and spinal cord decompression accidents.

In the etiological assessment of MI secondary to post-VZV vasculitis, we emphasize the contribution of diffusion MRI and the search for intrathecal synthesis.

Even with a complete etiological workup, the cause may remain undetermined in a quarter of cases.

This is a rare but serious complication that requires appropriate management in both the acute and chronic phases. It can improve even at a distance from the acute episode, which is why these patients should be monitored clinically.

Although there are currently no recommendations for the treatment of MI, control of hemodynamic parameters by vasopressors, CSF drainage and thrombolysis within 6 hours of symptomatology onset would enable better management of MI. Other therapeutic trials are underway based on Nrf2 activation [55].

The main poor prognostic factors in our study were the extent of motor deficits in the first 24 hours and the lack of improvement after the acute phase, as well as advanced age and, of course, the severe and life-threatening nature of the underlying pathology.

In previous studies, other poor prognostic factors have been incriminated, such as female gender, the presence of vesico-sphincter disorders and proprioceptive impairment.

Involving as many neurology centers as possible would enable us to carry out a more extensive study, which would ensure greater legitimacy for our results, thanks to a larger sample of patients, but also in order to reach a therapeutic consensus, which has been a long time coming.

REFERENCES

1.   **de Seze**, M., et al, [Functional prognosis of paraplegia due to cord ischemia: a retrospective study of 23 patients]. Rev Neurol (Paris), 2003. 159(11): p. 103845.

2.   **Kumral**, E., et al, Spinal ischaemic stroke: clinical and radiological findings and short-term outcome. Eur J Neurol, 2011. 18(2): p. 232-9

3.   **Robertson**, C.E., et al, Recovery after spinal cord infarcts: long-term outcome in 115 patients. Neurology, 2012. 78(2): p. 114-21.

4.   **Nedeltchev**, K., et al, Long-term outcome of acute spinal cord ischemia syndrome. Stroke, 2004. 35(2): p. 560-5.

5.   **Cheng**, M.Y., et al, Spinal cord infarction in Chinese patients. Clinical features, risk factors, imaging and prognosis. Cerebrovasc Dis, 2008. 26(5): p. 502-8.

6.   **Struhal** W., et al, Clinical core symptoms of posterior spinal artery ischemia. Eur Neurol, 2011.65(4): p. 183-186

7.   **Novy**, J., et al, Spinal cord ischemia: clinical and imaging patterns, pathogenesis, and outcomes in 27 patients. Arch Neurol, 2006. 63(8): p. 111320.

8.   **Ogawa** K1, Suzuki Y2, Oishi M2, Kamei S2.Clinical study of 46 patients with lateral medullary infarction. Stroke Cerebrovasc Dis. 2015 May;24(5):1065-74.

9.   **New**, P.W. and C.L. Mc Farlane, Retrospective case series of outcomes following spinal cord infarction. Eur J Neurol, 2012. 19(9): p. 1207-12

10.   **Calabro RS**. et al. Pudendal nerve stimulation: A potential tool for neurogenic bowel dysfunction. Neurourol Urodyn, 2013. 9999: p 1-2.

11.   **Vargas MI**, Gariani J, Sztajzel R et al (2015) Spinal cord ischemia: practical imaging tips, pearls, and pitfalls. AJNR Am J Neuroradiol 36:825-830.

12.   **Wrigley PJ**, et al, Longstanding neuropathic pain after spinal cord injury is refractory to transcranial direct current stimulation: A randomized controlled trial. Pain, 2013. July 4.

13.   **Kister I**, Johnson E, Raz E, Babb J, Loh J, Shepherd TM. Specific MRI findings help distinguish acute transverse myelitis of neuromyelitis optica from spinal cord

infarction. Mult Scler Relat Disord. 2016; 9: 62-7.

14. **Vargasl** & B. M. A. Delattre2 & J. Botol & J. Gariani2 & A. Dhouib2 & A. Fitsiori & J. L. Dietemann. Advanced magnetic resonance imaging (MRI) techniques of the spine and spinal cord in children and adults. Insights Imaging. 2018 Jun 1. doi: 10.1007/s13244-018- 0626-1. [Epub ahead of print]

15. **Dogan VB** , et al. A case with angiographic demonstration of isolated anterior spinal artery occlusion. Ideggyogy Sz. 2018. Mar 30;71(3-04)

16. **Masson, C.,** et al, Spinal cord infarction: clinical and magnetic resonance imaging findings and short term outcome. J Neurol Neurosurg Psychiatry, 2004. 75(10): p. 1431-5.

17. **Naess**, H. and F. Romi, Comparing patients with spinal cord infarction and cerebral infarction: clinical characteristics, and short-term outcome. Vasc Health Risk Manag, 2011. 7: p. 497-502.

18. **Reisner** A, Gary MF, Chern JJ, Grattan-Smith JD et al. Spinal cord infarction following minor trauma in children: fibrocartilaginous embolism as a putative cause. J Neurosurg Pediatr, 2013. 11:445-450

19. **Lewis SJ,** Gray R, Holmes LM et al. Neurophysiological changes in deformity correction of adolescent idiopathic scoliosis with intraoperative skull-femoral traction, Spine. 2013; 6: 1627-1638

20. **Do-Dai,** D.D., et al, Magnetic resonance imaging of intramedullary spinal cord lesions: a pictorial review. Curr Probl Diagn Radiol, 2010. 39(4): p. 160-85.

21. **Buth J,** Harris PL, Hobo R, van Eps R, Cuypers P, Duijm L, Tielbeek X. Neurologic complications associated with endovascular repair of thoracic aortic pathology: incidence and risk factors. A study from the European Collaborators on Stent/Graft Techniques for Aortic Aneurysm Repair (EUROSTAR) registry. J Vasc Surg. 2007;46(6):1103-10.

22. **Hsu CY**, Cheng CY, Lee JD, Lee M, Huang YC, Wu CY, et al. Clinical features and outcomes of spinal cord infarction following vertebral artery dissection: a systematic review of the literature. Neurol Res. 2013;35(7):676-83. 20.

23. **Watts J,** Box GA, Galvin A, Van Tonder F, Trost N, Sutherland T.Magnetic resonance imaging of intramedullary spinal cord lesions: a pictorial review. J Med

Imaging Radiat Oncol. 2014 Oct;58(5):569-81

24.	**Chang CW**, Donovan DJ, Liem LK, O'Phelan KH, Green DM, Bassin S, et al. Surfers' myelopathy: a case series of 19 novice surfers with nontraumatic myelopathy. Neurology. 2012;79(22):2171-6. 25.

25.	**Thompson TP**, Pearce J, Chang G, Madamba J. Surfer's myelopathy. Spine. 2004;29(16):E353-6. 26.

26.	**Freedman BA**, Malone DG, Rasmussen PA, Cage JM, Benzel EC. Surfer's myelopathy: a rare form of spinal cord infarction in novice surfers: a systematic review. Neurosurgery. 2016;78(5):602-11.

27.	**Dillen WL,** et al. Surfer's myelopathy: A rare presentation in a teenage gymnast and review of the literature. J Clin Neurosci. 2018 (article in press)

28.	**Maria A**. Nagel et al, Update on Varicella Zoster Virus Vasculopathy Curr Infect Dis Rep. 2014 June ; 16(6): 407

29.	**Deena M**. Nasr, DO1,* Alejandro Rabinstein, MD et al. Spinal Cord Infarcts: Risk Factors, Management, and Prognosis. Curr Treat Options Neurol (2017) 19:28

30.	**Etgen T**, Hocherl C. Repeated early thrombolysis in cervical spinal cord ischemia. J Thromb Thrombolysis. 2016;42 (1):142-5.

31.	**Muller KI**, Steffensen LH, Johnsen SH. Thrombolysis in anterior spinal artery syndrome. BMJ Case Rep.2012;2012

32.	**Restrepo L**, Guttin JF. Acute spinal cord ischemia during aortography treated with intravenous thrombolytic therapy. Tex Heart Inst J. 2006;33(1):74-7.

33.	**Rain S**, Udding J, Broere D. Acute clinical worsening after steroid administration in cervical myelitis may reveal a subdural arteriovenous fistula. Case Rep Neurol. 2016;8(3):234-42.

34.	**Nasr DM,** Brinjikji W, Rabinstein AA, Lanzino G. Clinical outcomes following corticosteroid administration in patients with delayed diagnosis of spinal arteriovenous fistulas. J Neurointervent Surg. 2017 Jun;9(6):607-610

35.	**Sugiura J** ,Oshima H, AbeT, NaritaY, ArakiY, Fujimoto K, et al. The efficacy and risk of cerebrospinal fluid drainage for thoracoabdominal aortic aneurysm repair: a retrospective observational comparison between drainage and non-drainage dagger. Interactive cardiovascular and thoracic surgery. 2017 Apr 1;24(4):609-614

36.   **Pollock NW**, Buteau D. Updates in decompression illness. Emerg Med Clin North Am. 2017;35(2):301- 19.

37.   **Rubin MN,** Rabinstein AA. Vascular diseases of the spinal cord. Neurol Clin. 2013;31(1):153- 81

38.   **New PW**, Mc Farlane CL. Survival following spinal cord infarction. Spinal Cord. 2013;51(6):453-6.

39.   **Rigney L**, Cappelen-Smith C, Sebire D, Beran RG, Cordato D. Nontraumatic spinal cord ischaemic syndrome. J Clin Neurosci: Off J Neurosurg Soc Australasia. 2015;22(10):1544-9.

40.   **Sandhu HK**, et al. Risk of Mortality after Resolution of Spinal Mal perfusion in Acute Dissection. Ann Thorac Surg. 2018 Mar 17. pii: S0003-4975(18)30364-3. doi: 10.1016/j.athoracsur.2018.02.035. [Epub ahead of print]

41.   **Moulakakis KG**, et al. Spinal cord ischemia following elective endovascular repair of infrarenal aortic aneurysms: A systematic review. 2018 Jun 6. pii: S0890-5096(18)30417-5. doi: 10.1016/j.avsg.2018.03.042. [Epub ahead of print] Review.

42.   **Heldner MR**, Arnold M, Nedeltchev K, Gralla J, Beck J, Fischer U. Vascular diseases of the spinal cord: a review. Curr Treat Options Neurol. 2012 ;14(6):509-20. 44.

43.   **Romi F**, Naess H. Spinal cord infarction in clinical neurology: a review of characteristics and long-term prognosis in comparison to cerebral infarction. Eur Neurol. 2016;76(3-4):95-8.

44.   **Hanson SR**, Romi F, Rekand T, Naess H. Long-term outcome after spinal cord infarctions. Acta Neurol Scand. 2015;131(4):253-7.

45.   **Vuckovic A**, Gallardo VJF, Jarjees M, Fraser M, Purcell M. Prediction of central neuropathic pain in spinal cord injury based on EEG classifier. Clin Neurophysiol. 2018 May 23;129(8):1605-1617. doi: 10.1016/j.clinph.2018.04.750.[Epub ahead of print]

46.   **Finnerup NB**, et al, Lamotrigine in spinal cord injury pain: a randomized controlled trial. Pain, 2002. 96(3): p. 375-83.

47.   **Salvador** de la Barrera, S., et al, Spinal cord infarction: prognosis and recovery in a series of 36 patients. Spinal Cord, 2001. 39(10): p. 520-5.

48.   **Pelser**, H. and J. van Gijn, Spinal infarction. A follow-up study. Stroke, 1993. 24(6): p. 896-8.

49.   **Cheshire**, W.P., et al, Spinal cord infarction: etiology and outcome. Neurology,

1996. 47(2): p. 321-30.

50. **New**, P.W., et al, A population-based study comparing traumatic spinal cord injury and non-traumatic spinal cord injury using a national rehabilitation database. Spinal Cord, 2011. 49(3): p. 397-403.

51. **Scivoletto**, G., et al, Recovery following ischemic myelopathies and traumatic spinal cord lesions. Spinal Cord, 2011. 49(8): p. 897-902.

52. **Pouw**, M.H., et al, Is the outcome in acute spinal cord ischaemia different from that in traumatic spinal cord injury? A cross-sectional analysis of the neurological and functional outcome in a cohort of 93 paraplegics. Spinal Cord, 2011. 49(2): p. 307-12.

53. **Yokoyama**, O., et al, Paraplegia after aortic aneurysm repair versus traumatic spinal cord injury: functional outcome, complications, and therapy intensity of inpatient rehabilitation. Arch Phys Med Rehabil, 2006. 87(9): p. 1189-94.

54. **Léa chiche** et al. Spinal cord ischemia in Scheuermann disease: A report of three cases. 2017, 84: 345-348

55. **Wang L, et al.** Methane ameliorates spinal cord ischemia-reperfusion injury in rats: Antioxidant, anti-inflammatory and anti-apoptotic activity mediated by Nrf2 activation. Biol Med. 2017,103:69-86

SUMMARY

The Goal:

Medullary infarction (MI) is both serious and rare. Diagnosis is based on a suggestive clinical picture and magnetic resonance imaging (MRI). The main objectives of our study were to identify the rather rare etiologies of MI, to update the management of MI and to determine the prognostic elements and complications of MI.

Methods :

This is a retrospective study including all patients followed at the Neurology Department of CHU Habib Bourguiba-Sfax over a period of 23 years and 14 years at the Neurology Department of CHU Sahloul-Sousse in whom the diagnosis of MI was retained. We collected the clinical, para-clinical, therapeutic and evolutionary characteristics of all these patients.

Results :

MI frequently affects the lower part of the dorsal spinal cord. Our study highlighted rare etiologies of MI such as surfer's myelopathy, systemic lupus erythematosus and post-VZV vasculitis. In the etiological assessment of MI secondary to post-VZV vasculitis, we emphasize the contribution of diffusion MRI and the search for intrathecal synthesis. Treatment in our study was essentially etiological. Currently, treatment is based on control of hemodynamic parameters with vasopressors and CSF drainage. Thrombolysis has been reported in the literature within 6 hours of onset of symptoms.

We noted improvement in 66.66% of patients, even at a distance from the acute episode, prompting clinical follow-up of these patients. The main poor prognostic factors in our study were the extent of motor deficits during the first 24 hours and the absence of improvement after the acute phase, as well as advanced age and, of course, the severity of the underlying etiology. In previous studies, other factors were revealed, such as female gender, the presence of vesico- sphincter disorders and proprioceptive impairment.

Conclusion:

Diffusion MRI was the most effective means of retaining the diagnosis of MI. Even with a complete etiological work-up, the cause may remain undetermined in a quarter of cases. It is a rare but serious complication, requiring appropriate management in both the acute and chronic phases. Although there are currently no recommendations for the treatment of MI, therapeutic trials are progressing in thrombolysis, CSF drainage and the prescription of vasopressors.

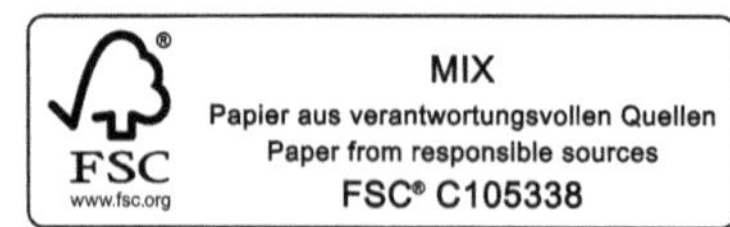

Printed by Books on Demand GmbH, Norderstedt / Germany